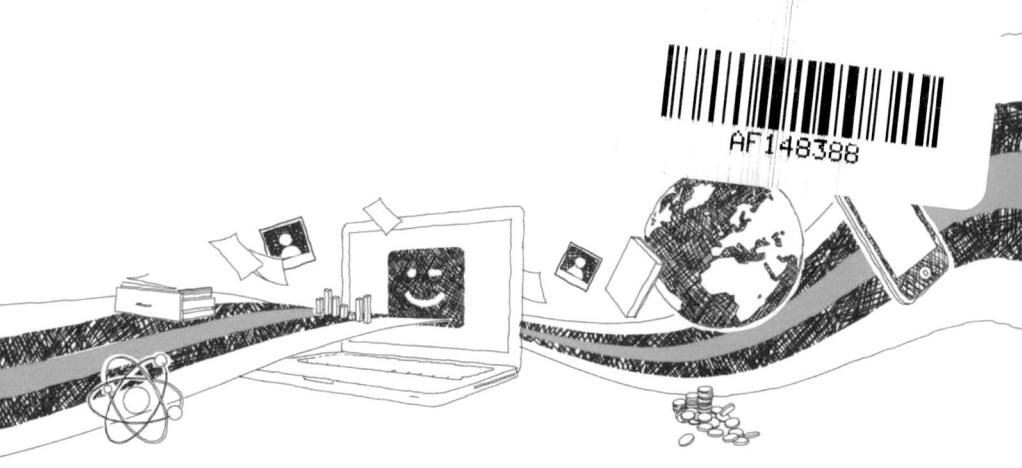

Bibliographic information published by the German National Library:

The German National Library lists this publication in the National Bibliography; detailed bibliographic data are available on the Internet at http://dnb.dnb.de .

Imprint:

Copyright © 2014 GRIN Verlag, Open Publishing GmbH
Print and binding: Books on Demand GmbH, Norderstedt Germany
ISBN: 9783668548817

This book at GRIN:

http://www.grin.com/en/e-book/377210/an-evidence-based-evaluation-of-a-hierarchical-model-of-memory

Haripriya Srinivasaraghavan

An Evidence-Based Evaluation of a Hierarchical Model of Memory

GRIN Publishing

GRIN - Your knowledge has value

Since its foundation in 1998, GRIN has specialized in publishing academic texts by students, college teachers and other academics as e-book and printed book. The website www.grin.com is an ideal platform for presenting term papers, final papers, scientific essays, dissertations and specialist books.

Visit us on the internet:

http://www.grin.com/

http://www.facebook.com/grincom

http://www.twitter.com/grin_com

Contents

Introduction   1

Hierarchical memory systems   1

Memory Prediction Framework   2

Evaluating the model – Predictions and Evidence   3

Implicit memory   4

Procedural learning   5

Semantic Memory   5

Episodic Memory   6

Discussion   8

Conclusion   8

References   9

An evidence based evaluation of a hierarchical model of memory

Introduction

Human memory is complex and multi-faceted with blurred boundaries shared with perception, thought, attention, control and consciousness. Many models of memory have been proposed over the years that attempt to address the systems, processes and mechanisms of memory. In this paper a hierarchical model of memory is discussed and is evaluated against its predictions in the face of experimental evidence in episodic, semantic, and implicit memory research from the fields of experimental psychology, cognitive neuroscience and animal neuroscience.

Hierarchical memory systems

There are many models that seek to explain biological memory. Unitary memory systems have been proposed where all functions of memory can be effectively achieved using a single set of laws or general principles, and they have been shown to account for some dissociations seen between recognition memory and repetition priming [Kinder and Shanks]. Unitary models have also been proposed based on the overarching similarities across regions in the neo-cortical substrate [Mountcastle].

But much experimental evidence has suggested a non-unitary memory model citing double dissociations, stochastic correlation and functional incompatibilities between single-shot learning, as seen in episodic memory, and habit or procedural learning. [Schachter, McClelland].

Apart from its functions, memory has also been studied based on the kind of organization. One such organization is a hierarchical memory model. Hierarchical models have been proposed to account for the operation of perceptual systems especially the visual system [Grossberg, Yuile] and in decision-making, cognition and executive control [Felleman], and using the Bayesian inference models [Friston, Hensen]. Bayesian models with their top-down probabilistic inference and the use of priors are inherently hierarchical.

Memory Prediction Framework

Jeff Hawkins proposed a memory based prediction framework [Hawkins] based on a hierarchical model of memory. This theory posits that the uniform arrangement of cortical tissue reflects a single algorithm that underlies all cortical information processing, where the basic principle is that of a hierarchy of cortical structures and a feedback loop that predicts and modulates the incoming perceptual stimuli. This theory goes beyond the memory functions alone, but uses memory as the underlying building block to create a cortical prediction framework that also involves the thalamus and the hippocampus.

The key concept of the framework is that bottom-up inputs trigger a series of partial matches in a hierarchy of recognition that generate top-down expectations from the upper layers. The predictions are spatio-temporal in nature. These expectations interact with the bottom-up inputs to predict future expected inputs. When bottom-up inputs match the top-down predictions at a particular level, that level recognizes the patterns and sends sparse 'labels' for these patterns up the hierarchy. This eliminates sending details to higher levels and facilitates the learning of higher-level features and invariant representations at higher levels. Higher levels predict more abstract or longer-term future sequences by matching partial sequences. But whenever there is insufficient matching at a particular level between the bottom-up inputs and the top-down predictions, more complete representations of the sequences are propagated. This leads to the higher layers looking for alternative interpretations for the input sequence, and results in modified predictions reaching the lower layers, which are again matched.

The layers at the very bottom of the hierarchy are the unimodal perceptual regions like vision. Higher regions learn more abstract or complex features that are relatively invariant and longer lasting compared to the lower level features. Unimodal regions lead to multimodal regions, association areas and finally to conceptual, semantic, language areas, each level representing more abstract or longer-term concepts. One can look at this as a Bayesian hierarchy, where top-down predictions represent Bayesian belief systems based on prior probabilities and bottom-up inputs are evaluated based on those beliefs. Only when a bottom-up input does not fit the top-down belief well, or when the top-down predictions are probabilistically weak, is the top-down belief system reevaluated. Alternately if the bottom-up inputs are unambiguous, then the system can reach a recognition result much faster, since the top-down predictions are not required to reach the level of activation required.

As one moves up the hierarchy, the representations show wider spatial and temporal receptive fields, increased temporal stability, and more abstraction. Also, sensory and motor hierarchies are intertwined so that actions can give rise to sensory expectations and sensory feedback can lead to motor actions. The thalamus and hippocampus are part of the proposed hierarchy, the former playing the role of a temporal delay line while the latter is thought to be at the summit of the hierarchy where unique patterns not captured by sufficient matches at lower layers, percolate to and are stored.

Temporal correlation is supposed to bind the patterns together. If one sees a picture while touching an object, these patterns can be tied together as a single pattern at higher levels because they co-occur in time. Some of these sub-patterns may have their representations and thus be propagated using sparse 'labels', but they are still tied together as objects or concepts co-occurring in an event or concept.

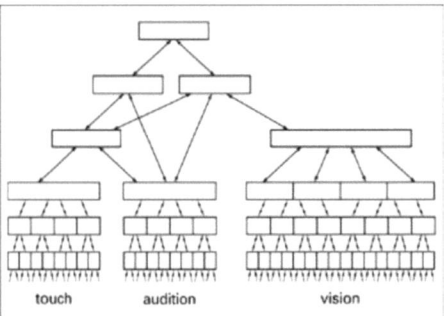

touch   audition   vision

Evaluating the model – Predictions and Evidence

According to this model, recognition and prediction are two sides of the same coin where prediction is an inherent part of perception and understanding and hence also of assimilation of new memories.

Some predictions of this model are:

1. One should find areas in the cortex that show enhanced activity in anticipation of a sensory event – In human fMRI studies activation patterns have been observed in the orbitofrontal cortex (OFC) during anticipation of a reward that are similar to the patterns seen during receipt of the reward [Kahnt].
2. A sudden flow of top-down activity should result when a new understanding emerges – when a visual illusion causes a change of interpretation, this should be accompanied by top-level changes while preserving permanency in lower level representations. This has been seen in Necker cube fMRI experiments, where activity is seen in non-visual regions during perceptual reversals. [Inui]

3

3. Faster vs. Slower: Perceptual recognition and recall tasks should be faster than conceptual tasks for the same inputs. This has been observed, where shallow depth of processing is associated with faster response times [Meijer]
4. There should be less activity in task specific regions when a pattern is recognized or expected. This is discussed in perceptual priming.
5. Increasingly complex patterns and features should be seen as one goes further away in the hierarchy from the sensory regions. More complex patterns and features are recognized by V4 and MT compared to V1 and V2 [Kamitani].
6. Unanticipated events should propagate up the hierarchy and completely novel events should reach top layers. The hippocampal and medial temporal lobe systems are considered to be at the very summit of this hierarchy and participate in the creation of episodic memories.
7. Representations and and complex features should move down the hierarchy with training: We will discuss this in procedural memory.
8. Invariant representations should be found in all cortical areas in the form of sparse cells that activate for a concept even when the perceptual inputs may differ. This is seen in parahippocampal place [O'Keefe] and grid cells [Fyhn] and in neurons that activate for the concept of Bill Clinton [Quiroga].

Implicit memory

Repetition suppression: Repetition suppression effects seen in perceptual priming experiments are consistent with prediction 2 in the previous section. Some of the proposed theories for repetition suppression – Bayesian explaining away [Henson, Friston], facilitation [James], and even sharpening [Desimone, Wiggs/Martin] theories - can coexist with or be explained by a hierarchical model. Facilitation predicts that the reduced activity seen in BOLD fMRI is because the activation shifts forward in time [Henson/Rugg], which could be due to reentrant modulation from higher areas. This can also be explained by higher-level predictions which when present disambiguate the input, speeding up the match. Sharpening can happen with priming because only matched 'labels' have to be sent instead of the entire pattern.

Priming and the Jacobi effect (false fame effect): One of the predictions of the hierarchical model is that if the bottom-up inputs are sufficiently strongly matched they can be recognized fast and emerge the winner among a set of potential patterns, even when top-level predictions for them don't match. So when a bottom-up pattern is predicted because it has been primed, the top-down layer only sees a winning pattern among a group of patterns without the reason of why it happened. This can lead to a misattribution of importance (false fame effect) [Jacoby], fluency heuristic [Whittlesea], or even misinterpretations [Gazzaniga]

Procedural learning

One of the predictions of the hierarchical model is that representations of complex features will move down the hierarchy with training. This would happen because the lower levels learn patterns not just from bottom-up stimuli but also from the prediction patterns that come top-down. When the same set of prediction patterns come through given the same bottom-up stimuli, these layers become better at predicting the patterns themselves without top-level hints. The effect of this is that the representations of these complex features effectively move down. Some examples of this effect are:

- When children learn to read, they read letter by letter but with practice they can directly read words or phrases. It has been shown that people read jumbled letters in a paragraph, without affecting recognition [Rayner][Keiigl].
- Chess players are able to remember complex board positions faster and better than novice players [Fernand/Simon]. Similarly an expert in a particular field is able to deal in higher-level constructs and concepts in that field at a much faster pace than someone who is a novice in that field.

Semantic Memory

Semantic memory is the memory for the general knowledge about the world. There are modal and amodal theories of how knowledge is represented. In the modal view, it is argued that semantic knowledge is tightly tied to the modalities it was acquired from [Barsolou], while amodal theories argue that pure semantic knowledge representations exist disconnected from their perceptual representations. But both models can coexist with distributed and hierarchical representation of knowledge. [Damasio] proposed a convergence zone framework, which proposes a hierarchy of association areas integrating modality specific information. When one assumes a set of hierarchies rather than a single hierarchy, the resulting structure assumes the properties of a highly connected network with a set of hubs, and where memory and thought can be seen as navigation or exploration of that network [Baroncelli].

Specific vs. general categorization: In experimental evidence [Rogers/Patterson] gathered from patients with semantic dementia it has been observed that the memory for specifics or exemplar features (a hump for a camel) is lost but some ability to recognize the general category remains intact (the patients are still able to recognize an animal). This can be explained reasonably well by a hierarchical model - in the absence of the representations available at a specific level, patterns cannot be sufficiently matched at that level, but they can still be matched at a higher, more invariant super-level. A hierarchical model can also explain why normal controls are faster to recognize objects at the basic level (dog rather than animal) –

the concept of a dog is matched much lower in the hierarchy compared to an animal when traversed using the perceptual cues.

The anterior shift seen in fMRI experiments when thinking about a concept compared to experiencing it might suggest a representation of concepts which can then be translated into modal patterns down a hierarchy.

Spreading activation model and transfer appropriate processing: The spreading activation model and the theory of transfer appropriate processing also make sense if one thinks of a hierarchical organization of semantic concepts, which are then traversed using different levels of cues. Depending on which level of cue finds a strong match (at a visual level, verbal level or at a conceptual level), different layers in the hierarchy becomes closer, and thus activate first. When one sees flat grass rather than rolled grass, the concept of 'roots' matches or activates more strongly [Barsalou].

Episodic memory

Episodic memory has long been looked at as the stumbling block to a unified memory model, because single-shot learning of episodes seems to be at cross-purposes to procedural learning.

The hierarchical model predicts that episodic memories are captured when patterns percolate up to the top of the hierarchy. Events can percolate up due to a variety of reasons.

- In any attended event, while a subset of the events might be pattern-matched, the uniqueness of the entire temporally correlated sequence of multi-modal patterns can send it all the way up the hierarchy. (When one goes to a new city, some aspects are new and are remembered along with the other expected patterns to make a unique event).
- The emotional strength or the attention associated with an event can provide strong modulation, and patterns of similar strength may not be found, so the entire pattern can be remembered at the top as something important. (A person may have dined in the same restaurant multiple times, but the first dinner with a girlfriend will be remembered uniquely).

It also predicts that patterns once unique will move down the hierarchy, with repeated exposure to same or similar patterns, to form generalized abstracted patterns – since components of unique memories can still facilitate a match at lower levels. This also accounts for 'semanticization' of memories with the passage of time, and reduction of hippocampal dependency. Generalization can also be the role of consolidation, viewed as a combination of reinstatement (replay) and pattern relearning. This is similar to the development of expertise in procedural learning.

Similarity between memory types

When patterns of matched activations are strong enough, they quickly percolate up with feature 'labels' and are matched with episodic traces at the top. This results in *recollection* of contextual features.

When lower patterns are not strongly matched, top-down predictions can select patterns that are strong enough. Depending on the accuracy and strength of these patterns episodic reconstruction can be attempted, but when a match happens that misses contextual features, *familiarity* is reported.

When multiple patterns are potentially matched bottom-up, only the winners percolate up. While only the winners capture conscious attention the other patterns can still be learned at the lower levels leading to *implicit memory* or priming. This is independent of the higher regions and can account for the dissociation found in amnesic patients.

A single computational model simulating recognition and implicit memory was also proposed by [McClelland]. It is possible that priming, familiarity and recollection are just different stages in a memory continuum modulated by conscious selection and attention.

Episodic and semantic memories may also be similar in their reinstatement or reenactment processes during consolidation and retrieval [Damasio] [Nadal/Moscovitch], which are inherently hierarchical, as higher-level concepts are mapped to lower level patterns in both cases.

Memory accuracy and errors: The prediction that episodic memory trace ties together semantic concepts stored in lower layers also accounts for errors in eye-witness testimony [Loftus], DRM [Roediger/McDermott] experiments, and script-based memories [Bower]. This suggests that episodic memory is not a faithful copy of the event, but is stored using generic representations and context, and that predictions play a role in the patterns observed.

Single-shot vs. repetitive learning: Episodic memory is thought to be single shot, but this is not always true. Memories are remembered with varying level of details, and sometimes there is only a vague sense of familiarity without sufficient contextual details. Many memories are vague, inaccurate [Loftus] or incomplete (Script or schema based memories [Starasina]). Episodic learning happens only for less complex stimuli, and where motor or verbatim outputs are not learning outcomes. Procedural learning, song learning and language learning on the other hand involve multiple sessions.

When a new stimulus is sufficiently complex or does not involve a known schema, it may take more time for learning to occur [van Kusteren] Remembering the name of a song is easier for a single-shot learning system than learning a new song, which involves multiple trials because of the complexity and the novelty.

Discussion

Previous sections suggest that a hierarchical memory model can account for many empirical results across semantic, episodic and implicit memory literature. While not conclusive or exhaustive this is a promising area to pursue further. At the same time, the hierarchical model may also be too generic or abstract to actually explain all major results in memory research. This is because it seems to fit almost any observation, given its lack of specificity, and thus has the danger of being non-falsifiable. Claiming that memory uses a hierarchical model is not very different or more specific than claiming that memory uses an interconnected set of neurons. The model has to be made more specific, which should then be tested using simulation and experimentation.

It is also not very clear that there is a single uniform algorithm even though a hierarchical structure might explain the evidence. This is particularly true with episodic memory which might comprise of different neural structures or algorithms compared to the rest of the hierarchy. There is neural evidence that the hippocampus is anatomically different from the rest of the cortex. So it is fairly certain that there is difference in functionality as well. It is not required that different types of patterns – temporal patterns, is-a pattern, collections) are all learned using the same algorithms. Different types of networks such as attractor networks and winner-takes-all networks have been shown to exist in the brain. There could be a small set of algorithmic building blocks rather than just one to account for the complexity of the brain and memory.

Finally, memory cannot be viewed in isolation. There have to be interconnected explanations for phenomena such as attention, emotion and consciousness that should work in tandem with memory in an overarching theory, before it can explain how memory works.

Conclusion

A hierarchical system of memory can be shown to account for many findings in memory literature. This opens up the possibility that the research on memory, thought and perception might benefit from further study into this model, by making the model more specific, simulating and testing its predictions.

Submitted by
Name: Haripriya Srinivasaraghavan, Date: 12/08/2014

References

1. Kinder, Annette, and David R. Shanks. "Neuropsychological dissociations between priming and recognition: A single-system connectionist account." *Psychological Review* 110, no. 4 (2003): 728.

2. Mountcastle, Vernon. "An organizing principle for cerebral function: the unit model and the distributed system." (1978).

3. Schacter, Daniel L., C-Y. Peter Chiu, and Kevin N. Ochsner. "Implicit memory: A selective review." *Annual review of neuroscience* 16, no. 1 (1993): 159-182.

4. McClelland, James L., Bruce L. McNaughton, and Randall C. O'Reilly. "Why there are complementary learning systems in the hippocampus and neocortex: insights from the successes and failures of connectionist models of learning and memory." *Psychological review* 102, no. 3 (1995): 419.

5. Grossberg S. *Towards a Unified Theory of Neocortex: Laminar Cortical Circuits for Vision and Cognition.* Vol. 165. 2007.

6. Friston, Karl J., Daniel E. Glaser, Richard NA Henson, S. Kiebel, Christophe Phillips, and John Ashburner. "Classical and Bayesian inference in neuroimaging: applications." *Neuroimage* 16, no. 2 (2002): 484-512.

7. Hawkins, Jeff, and Sandra Blakeslee. *On intelligence.* Macmillan, 2007.

8. Felleman, D. J., and D. C. Van Essen. "Distributed Hierarchical Processing in the Primate Cerebral Cortex," Cerebral Cortex, vol. 1 (January/February 1991): pp. 1–47

9. Gotts, S. J., Chow, C. C., & Martin, A. (2012). Repetition Priming and Repetition Suppression: A Case for Enhanced Efficiency Through Neural Synchronization. *Cognitive Neuroscience*, 3(3-4), 227–237. doi:10.1080/17588928.2012.670617

10. Inui T, Tanaka S, Okada T, Nishizawa S, Katayama M, Konishi J. Neural substrates for depth perception of the Necker cube: A functional magnetic resonance imaging study in human subjects. Neuroscience Letters. 2000;282:145–148.

11. Kahnt, Thorsten, Jakob Heinzle, Soyoung Q. Park, and John-Dylan Haynes. "The neural code of reward anticipation in human orbitofrontal cortex." *Proceedings of the National Academy of Sciences* 107, no. 13 (2010): 6010-6015.

12. Kamitani, Yukiyasu, and Frank Tong. "Decoding the visual and subjective contents of the human brain." *Nature neuroscience* 8, no. 5 (2005): 679-685.

13. Meijer, Willemien A., Renate HM de Groot, Pascal WM van Gerven, Martin PJ van Boxtel, and Jelle Jolles. "Level of processing and reaction time in young and middle-aged adults and the effect of education." *European Journal of Cognitive Psychology* 21, no. 2-3 (2009): 216-234.

14. O'Keefe, John, and Neil Burgess. "Geometric determinants of the place fields of hippocampal neurons." *Nature* 381, no. 6581 (1996): 425-428.
15. Fyhn M, Molden S, Witter MP, Moser EI, Moser M-B. 2004. Spatial representation in the entorhinal cortex. *Science* 305:1258–64
16. Quiroga, R. Quian, Leila Reddy, Gabriel Kreiman, Christof Koch, and Itzhak Fried. "Invariant visual representation by single neurons in the human brain." *Nature* 435, no. 7045 (2005): 1102-1107.
17. Henson, R. (2003). Neuroimaging studies of priming. Progress in Neurobiology, 70(1), 53–81.
18. James, T. W., Humphrey, G. K., Gati, J. S., Menon, R. S., & Goodale, M. A. (2000). The effects of visual object prim- ing on brain activation before and after recognition. Current Biology, 10, 1017–1024.
19. Desimone, R. (1996). Neural mechanisms for visual memory and their role in attention. Proceedings of the National Academy of Sciences of the United States of America, 93, 13494–13499.
20. Wiggs, C. L., & Martin, A. (1998). Properties and mechan- isms of perceptual priming. Current Opinion in Neurobiology, 8, 227–233
21. Henson, R. N. A., and M. D. Rugg. "Neural response suppression, haemodynamic repetition effects, and behavioural priming." *Neuropsychologia* 41, no. 3 (2003): 263-270.
22. Jacoby, Larry L., Vera Woloshyn, and Colleen Kelley. "Becoming famous without being recognized: Unconscious influences of memory produced by dividing attention." *Journal of experimental psychology: General* 118, no. 2 (1989): 115.
23. Whittlesea, Bruce WA, and Jason P. Leboe. "The heuristic basis of remembering and classification: fluency, generation, and resemblance." *Journal of Experimental Psychology: General* 129, no. 1 (2000): 84.
24. Gazzaniga, Michael S. *Split Brain*. Insta-Tape, 1973.
25. Kersten, Daniel, Pascal Mamassian, and Alan Yuille. "Object perception as Bayesian inference." *Annu. Rev. Psychol.* 55 (2004): 271-304.
26. Rayner, Keith, Sarah J. White, Rebecca L. Johnson, and Simon P. Liversedge. "Raeding Wrods With Jubmled Lettres There Is a Cost." *Psychological science* 17, no. 3 (2006): 192-193.
27. Kliegl, Reinhold, Antje Nuthmann, and Ralf Engbert. "Tracking the mind during reading: the influence of past, present, and future words on fixation durations." *Journal of experimental psychology: General* 135, no. 1 (2006): 12.
28. Gobet, Fernand, and Herbert A. Simon. "Recall of random and distorted chess positions: Implications for the theory of expertise." *Memory & cognition* 24, no. 4 (1996): 493-503.

29. Tulving, Endel. "Episodic and semantic memory 1." *Organization of Memory. London: Academic* 381 (1972): e402.
30. Barsalou, Lawrence W., W. Kyle Simmons, Aron K. Barbey, and Christine D. Wilson. "Grounding conceptual knowledge in modality-specific systems." *Trends in cognitive sci*
31. Damasio, Antonio R., and Hannah Damasio. "Cortical systems for retrieval of concrete knowledge: The convergence zone framework." *Large-scale neuronal theories of the brain* (1994): 61-74
32. Networks in Cognitive Science, Andrea Baronchelli, Ramon Ferrer-i-Cancho, Romualdo Pastor-Satorras, Nick Chater, Morten H. Christiansen, Reviews, Cell Press, 2013
33. Rogers, T. T. & Patterson, K. Object categorization: reversals and explanations of the basic-level advantage. *J. Exp. Psychol. Gen.*, 136, 451–469 (2007).
34. Staresina, B. P., Gray, J. C., & Davachi, L. (2009). Event congruency enhances episodic memory encoding through semantic elaboration and relational binding. Cerebral Cortex, 19(5), 1198-1207. doi:10.1093/cercor/bhn165
35. Damasio, A.R. (1989) Time-locked multiregional retroactivation: a systems-level proposal for the neural substrates of recall and recognition. Cognition 33, 25–62
36. Barsalou, Lawrence W. "Grounded cognition." *Annu. Rev. Psychol.* 59 (2008): 617-645.
37. Loftus, Elizabeth F., and Jacqueline E. Pickrell. "The formation of false memories." *Psychiatric annals* 25, no. 12 (1995): 720-725.
38. Bower, Gordon H., John B. Black, and Terrence J. Turner. "Scripts in memory for text." *Cognitive psychology* 11, no. 2 (1979): 177-220.
39. van Kesteren, Marlieke TR, Dirk J. Ruiter, Guillén Fernández, and Richard N. Henson. "How schema and novelty augment memory formation." *Trends in neurosciences* 35, no. 4 (2012): 211-219.

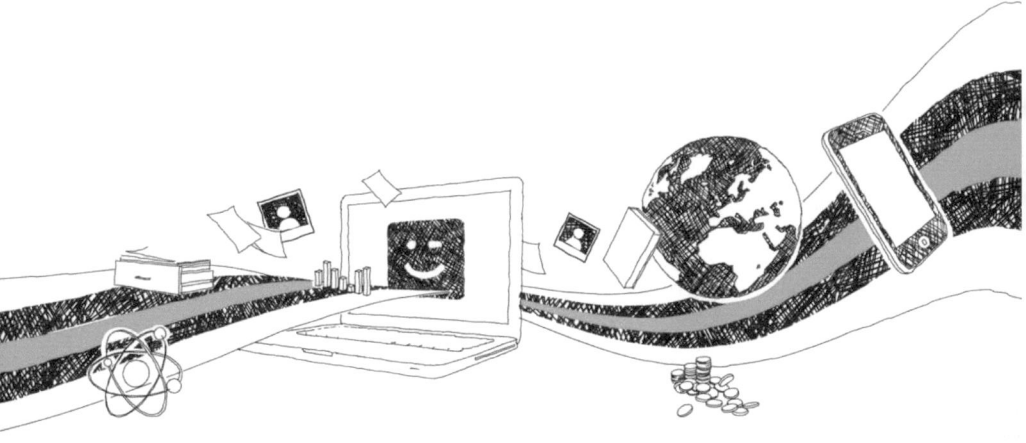
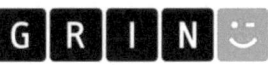